FAVORITES MEXICAN RECIPES.

A FLAVOR-BURSTING FIESTA OF DISHES

By Delia Suarez

TABLE OF CONTENTS

FLAVORFUL MEXICAN MOLE 7

EASY MEXICAN FRIED CHICKEN 9

CHICKEN KABOBS MEXICANA 11

MEXICAN BEAN PIE 13

FANTASTIC MEXICAN DIP 15

MEXICAN BROWNIES 17

MEXICAN CORNBREAD SALAD 19

MEXICAN PIZZA 21

MEXICAN PIZZA 1 23

RICH MEXICAN CORN 25

MEXICAN CORN 27

CORNY MEXICAN SALAD 28

MOM'S HOT MEXICAN SALAD 29

MEXICAN STYLE CORNBREAD 31

MEXICAN CORNBREAD II 33

MEXICAN TURKEY 34

SMOTHERED MEXICAN LASAGNA 35

MEXICAN CASSEROLE 37

AUSTIN MARGARITA (AKA MEXICAN MARTINI) 39

MEXICAN WHITE RICE 41

SCRUMPTIOUS 5-LAYER MEXICAN DIP 43

MEXICAN LASAGNA CHIP DIP 44

MEXICAN LASAGNA 46

MEXICAN LASAGNA (1) 49

MEXICAN LASAGNA (2) 51

MEXICAN LASAGNA ROLLUPS 53

MEXICAN EGG ROLLS 56

MEXICAN ORANGE CHICKEN 58

ABSOLUTE MEXICAN CORNBREAD 60

MOM'S MEXICAN CORNBREAD 62

MEXICAN STYLE MEATBALLS 64

BASIC MEXICAN GUACAMOLE 67

CAMPBELL'S KITCHEN MEXICAN STROGANOFF 69

CREAMY MEXICAN DIP 71

EASY MEXICAN CASSEROLE 72

MEXICAN SALSA II 74

MEXICAN POSOLE STEW 75

CALDO DE RES (MEXICAN BEEF SOUP) 77

CHOCOLATE MEXICAN WEDDING COOKIES 79

GROUND BEEF MEXICAN STYLE 81

HOT MEXICAN SPINACH DIP 83

MEXICAN-STYLE GOULASH 85

MEXICAN BRUNCH TORTILLAS 86

MEXICAN SPINACH DIP 88

MEXICAN GRILLED CHICKEN 91

MEXICAN CHICKEN AND BLACK BEAN SALAD 92

MEXICAN WEDDING CAKES II 94

MEXICAN MEAT LOAF 95

MEXICAN PINTO BEANS 96

MEXICAN SALMON 98

MEXICAN CORN SALAD 100

MEXICAN HOT DIP 101

Flavorful Mexican Mole

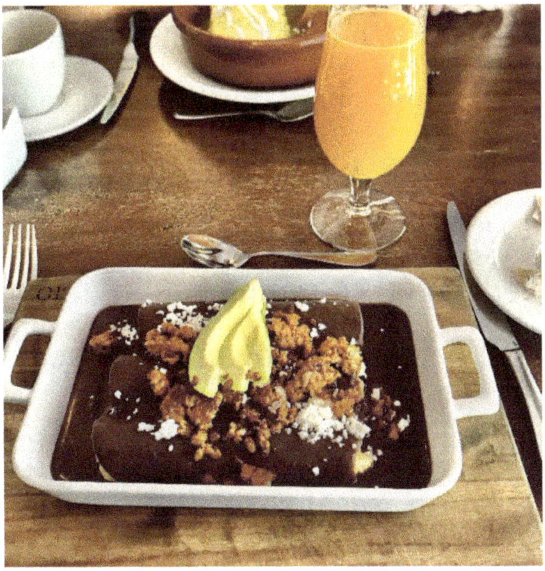

Ingredients

- 20 roma (plum) tomatoes 8 fresh jalapeño peppers
- 1/4 cup crushed walnuts
- 1/3 cup sesame seeds
- 1/4 cup raisins
- 3 ounces bittersweet chocolate, melted
- 2 tablespoons minced garlic
- 1-quart vegetable stock

Directions

Preheat the oven broiler. Place the tomatoes and jalapeno peppers on a baking sheet, and broil for about 5 minutes, turning once, until they have begun to scorch on all sides. Remove from heat. Transfer the peppers to a bowl, and cover tightly with plastic wrap until cooled, about 15 minutes. Slip the skins off the peppers, slit peppers open, and remove the seeds.

In a blender or food processor, blend the tomatoes, peppers, walnuts, sesame seeds, raisins, chocolate, and garlic.

Heat a skillet sprayed with cooking spray over medium-high heat. Cook and stir the blended mixture in the skillet until heated through.

Return the mixture to the blender. Blend in enough of the vegetable stock to make a slightly thick sauce. Cool, and store in the refrigerator until ready to use.

Easy Mexican Fried Chicken

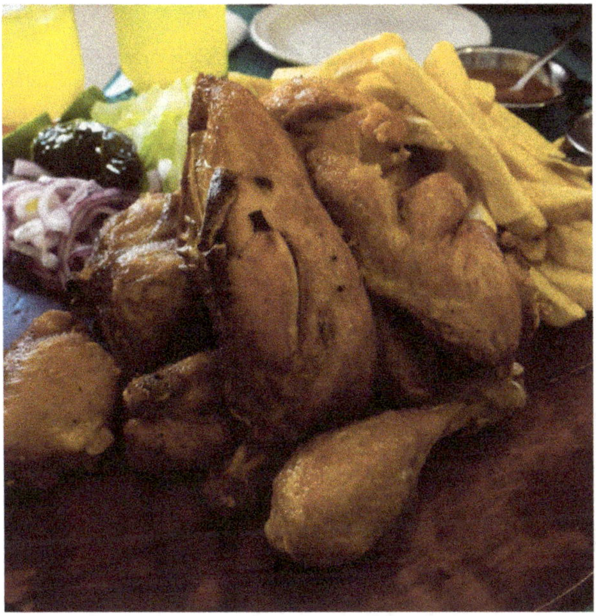

Ingredients

- 4 skinless, boneless chicken breast halves
- 1-quart buttermilk
- 2 (1.25 ounce) packages taco seasoning mix
- 3 tablespoons olive oil
- 1 1/2 cups all-purpose flour

Directions

In a resealable plastic bag, combine the chicken, buttermilk, and 1 packet of taco seasoning. Seal and shake to mix together.

Refrigerate and let marinate overnight.

In a large skillet, heat the olive oil over medium-low heat. Mix flour and the other packet of taco seasoning in a shallow dish or plate. Remove chicken from refrigerator and remove chicken from marinade. Discard marinade.

Coat chicken with flour mixture and fry in skillet until cooked through and juices run clear 15 to 20 minutes.

Chicken Kabobs Mexicana

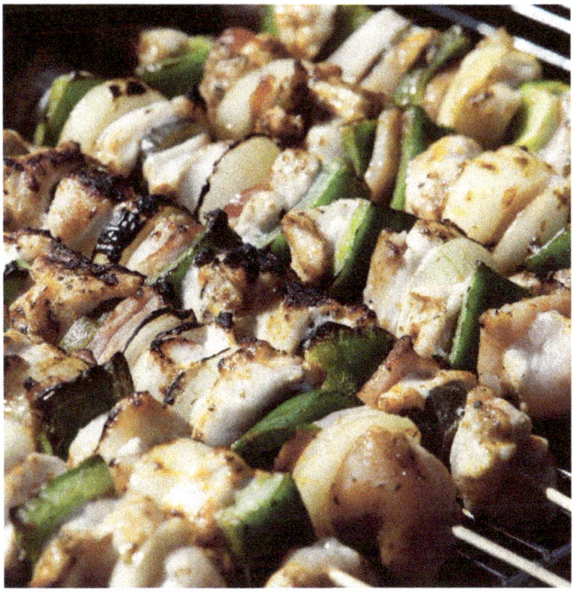

Ingredients

2 tablespoons olive oil

- 1 teaspoon ground cumin
- 2 tablespoons chopped fresh cilantro
- 1 lime, juiced
- salt and ground black pepper to taste
- 2 skinless, boneless chicken breast halves - cut into 1-inch cubes
- 1 small zucchini, cut into 1/2-inch slices

- 1 onion, cut into wedges, and separated
- 1 red bell pepper, cut into 1-inch pieces
- 10 cherry tomatoes

Directions

In a shallow dish, mix together olive oil, cumin, chopped cilantro, and lime juice. Season with salt and pepper. Add chicken and mix well. Cover, and refrigerate for at least one hour.

Preheat grill for high heat.

Thread chicken, zucchini, onion, red bell pepper, and tomatoes onto skewers.

Brush grill with oil and arrange skewers on the hot grate. Cook for approximately 10 minutes, or until chicken is cooked through, turning to cook evenly.

Mexican Bean Pie

Ingredients

- 1 (15 ounce) can black beans, drained and rinsed
- 1 (15 ounce) can pinto beans, drained
- 1 (16 ounce) can refried beans
- 1 (2 ounce) can sliced black olives
- 1/2 (15.25 ounce) can whole kernel corn, drained
- 1/2 cup chopped green bell pepper
- 1 jalapeno pepper, seeded and minced
- 1 tablespoon ground cumin
- 1 tablespoon chili powder ground black pepper to taste
- 5 (10 inch) whole wheat tortillas
- 1 1/2 cups shredded Cheddar cheese
- 1/2 cup salsa (optional)
- 1/2 cup sour cream (optional)

Directions

Preheat oven to 350 degrees F (175 degrees C). Lightly grease a 10-inch round cake pan or springform pan.

In a large saucepan over medium-high heat, mix black beans, pinto beans, refried beans, olives, corn, bell pepper, and jalapeno pepper. Season with cumin, chili powder, and black pepper. Cook and stir until thickened, about 10 minutes.

Lay one tortilla flat on the bottom of the prepared baking pan. Spread 1/4 of the bean mixture on the tortilla. Sprinkle 1/4 cup Cheddar cheese lightly over the bean mixture. Repeat layering, ending with a tortilla. Top with remaining Cheddar cheese.

Bake 20 minutes in the preheated oven. Allow to cool slightly before serving. Serve with salsa and sour cream for garnish.

Fantastic Mexican Dip

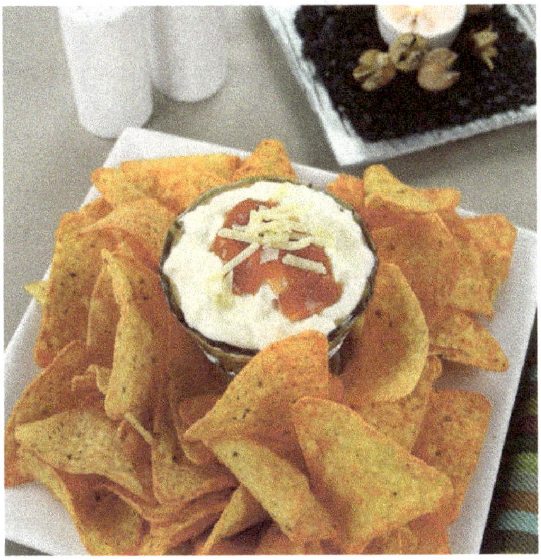

Ingredients

- 2 pounds lean ground beef 1 (16 ounce) jar taco sauce
- 1 (16 ounce) container sour cream
- 1 (8 ounce) package cream cheese, softened
- 1 (1 ounce) package taco seasoning mix
- 1 (16 ounce) package shredded Cheddar cheese
- 1 cup shredded lettuce
- 1 tomato, cubed
- 2 green onions, sliced
- 1 (2 ounce) can sliced black olives, drained

Directions

Crumble ground beef in a large, deep skillet. Cook over medium-high heat until evenly brown. Drain, mix in the taco sauce, and set aside.

In a large bowl, mix the sour cream, cream cheese, and taco seasoning mix. Spread the mixture into a medium serving dish.

Layer the sour cream mixture with beef mixture, Cheddar cheese, and lettuce. Top with tomato, green onions, and black olives.

Mexican Brownies

Ingredients

- 1 1/2 cups unsalted butter
- 3 cups white sugar
- 6 eggs
- 1 tablespoon vanilla extract
- 1 1/4 cups unsweetened cocoa powder
- 1 1/2 cups all-purpose flour
- 1 3/4 teaspoons ground Mexican cinnamon
- 1/2 teaspoon ground pequin chile pepper
- 3/4 teaspoon kosher salt
- 3/4 teaspoon baking powder

Directions

Preheat oven to 350 degrees F (175 degrees C). Line a 12x15-inch baking pan with parchment paper, leaving about 3 inches of paper overhanging 2 sides to use as handles.

Place the butter in a microwave-safe bowl and cook on Medium until the butter is about half melted, about 1 minute. Mash the butter with sugar until well combined, and stir in eggs one at a time, incorporating each one before adding the next. Mix in vanilla extract.

Sift the cocoa, flour, cinnamon, pequin pepper, salt, and baking powder into a bowl. Sprinkle in any salt caught in the sifter. Mix the flour mixture into the butter mixture, stirring to blend well, and pour the batter into the prepared baking pan.

Bake in the preheated oven until a toothpick inserted into the center comes out with moist crumbs, 20 to 25 minutes. Let cool in the pan and use parchment paper handles to remove the brownies for slicing.

Mexican Cornbread Salad

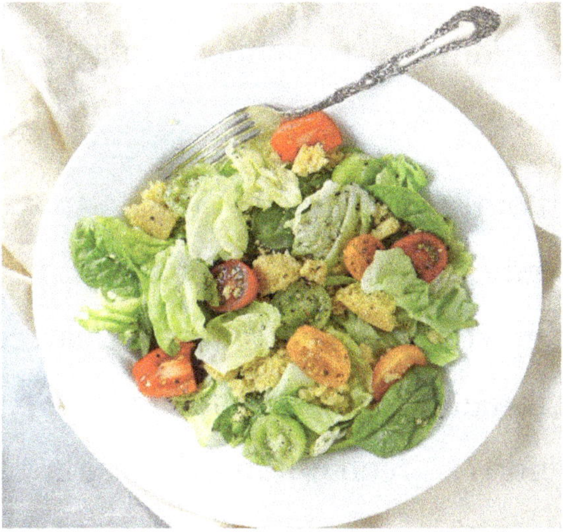

Ingredients

- 1 (8.5 ounce) package dry cornbread mix
- 1 (4 ounce) can chopped green chile peppers
- 2 (16 ounce) cans pinto beans, drained
- 1 (16 ounce) bottle Ranch-style salad dressing
- 1 green bell pepper, chopped
- 2 (15.25 ounce) cans whole kernel corn, drained
- 2 tomatoes, chopped
- 1 (3 ounce) can bacon bits
- 8 ounces shredded Cheddar cheese
- 1 green onions

Directions

Prepare cornbread mix according to package directions, adding green chiles. Set aside, allow to cool and crumble.

Place half of the cornbread at the bottom of a large bowl. Evenly layer with 1 can of beans, 1 cup salad dressing, 1/2 chopped bell pepper, 1 can corn, 1 chopped tomato, 1/2 jar bacon bits, 1/2 package cheese, and 1/2 green onions. Repeat layers in the same order using remaining ingredients, beginning with crumbled cornbread.

Cover, refrigerate 2 hours, and serve chilled.

Mexican Pizza

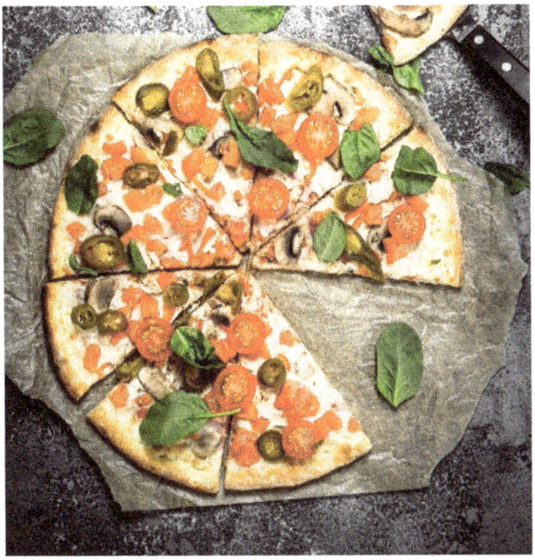

Ingredients

- 1/2 (16 ounce) can spicy fat-free refried beans
- 1 cup salsa, divided
- 1 (12 inch) prebaked Italian pizza crust
- 2 cups shredded hearts of romaine lettuce
- 3 medium green onions, thinly sliced
- 1/4 cup ranch dressing
- 1/4 cup crumbled tortilla chips
- 1 cup shredded pepper Jack or Monterey Jack cheese

Directions

Adjust oven rack to lowest position, and heat oven to 450 degrees. Mix beans and 1/2 cup salsa in a medium bowl. Place crust on a cookie sheet then spread the bean mixture over crust. Bake until it's crisp and warm, about 10 minutes.

Remove from oven, top with lettuce, green onions, and dollop with the remaining salsa. Drizzle (or, if the dressing has an easy-pour top, squirt) dressing over pizza. Top with chips and cheese, then return to the oven and bake until the cheese melts, about 2 minutes longer. Cut into 6 slices and serve.

Mexican Pizza 1

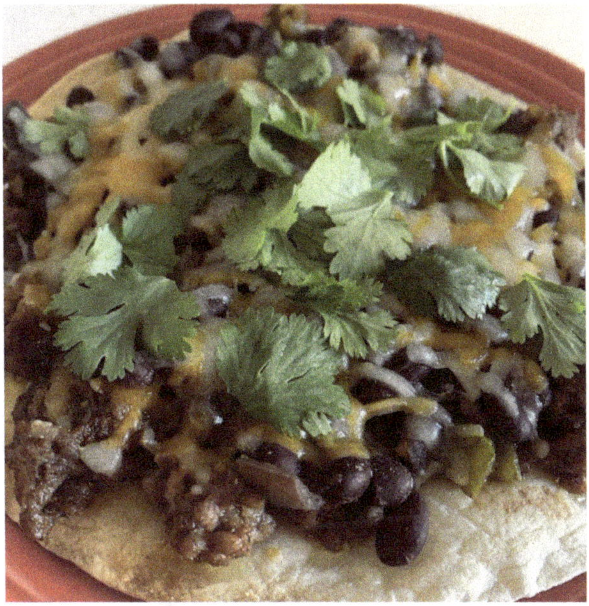

Ingredients

- 2 (8 ounce) cans refrigerated crescent rolls
- 1 (8 ounce) package cream cheese, softened
- 1 cup sour cream
- 1 pound ground beef
- 1 (1.25 ounce) package taco seasoning
- 1 (2.25 ounce) can sliced ripe olives, drained
- 1 medium tomato, chopped
- 3/4 cup shredded Cheddar cheese

- 3/4 cup shredded mozzarella cheese
- 1 cup shredded lettuce

Directions

Unroll crescent roll dough and place in an ungreased 15-in. x 10-in. x 1-in. baking pan. Flatten dough to fit the pan, sealing seams, and perforations. Bake at 375 degrees F for 8-10 minutes or until light golden brown; cool. In a small bowl, blend cream cheese and sour cream with a wire whisk; spread over crust. Chill 30 minutes.

Meanwhile, in a skillet, brown beef; drain. Stir in taco seasoning. Add water according to package directions and simmer for 5 minutes, stirring occasionally. Spread over cream cheese layer. Top with olives, tomato, cheeses, and lettuce. Cut into serving-size pieces. Serve immediately or refrigerate.

Rich Mexican Corn

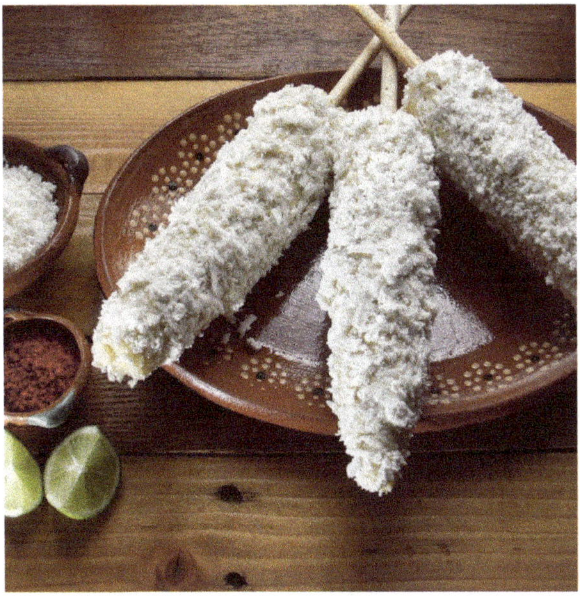

Ingredients

- 1 (8 ounce) package cream cheese
- 1/2 cup butter
- 1/2 cup milk
- 1 (16 ounce) package frozen corn
- 1 red bell pepper, diced
- 8 fresh jalapeno peppers, diced

Directions

Preheat oven to 350 degrees F (175 degrees C).

In a saucepan over medium-low heat, melt the cream cheese and butter, and mix with the milk until smooth and bubbly.

In a medium casserole dish, mix the frozen corn, red bell pepper, and jalapeno peppers. Pour in the cream cheese mixture and toss to coat.

Bake 35 to 45 minutes in the preheated oven until bubbly and lightly brown.

Mexican Corn

Ingredients

- 2 (15.25 ounce) cans whole kernel corn, drained
- 1 (8 ounce) package cream cheese
- 1/4 cup butter
- 10 jalapeno peppers, chopped
- 1 teaspoon garlic salt

Directions

In a medium saucepan, combine corn, cream cheese, butter, jalapeno peppers, and garlic salt. Cook over medium heat for about 10 minutes or until heated through, constantly stirring after cream cheese begins to melt.

Corny Mexican Salad

Ingredients

- 2 (15 ounce) cans black beans, rinsed and drained
- 1 (11 ounce) can Mexicorn, drained
- 1 medium tomato, chopped
- 1 medium ripe avocado, peeled and cubed
- 1/2 cup chopped onion
- 1/2 cup vegetable oil
- 1/4 cup red wine vinegar
- 1/2 teaspoon salt
- 1/2 teaspoon hot pepper sauce
- Tortilla chips

Directions

In a bowl, combine the beans, corn, tomato, avocado, and onion. In a small bowl, whisk the oil, vinegar, salt, and hot pepper sauce; pour over bean mixture and toss to coat. Serve with tortilla chips if desired.

Mom's Hot Mexican Salad

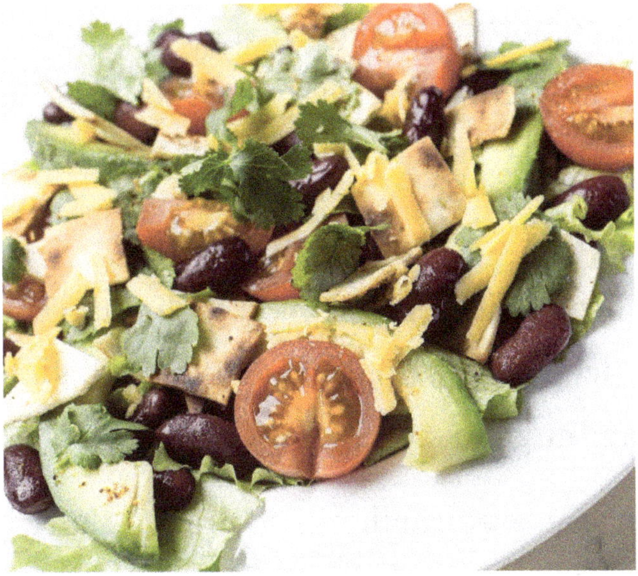

Ingredients

- 1 1/2 pounds lean ground beef
- 1 onion, diced
- 1 green bell pepper, diced
- 1 tablespoon garlic powder
- 1 tablespoon ground cumin
- 1-pound processed cheese food (e.g., Velveeta), cubed
- 1 (4 ounce) can diced green chiles
- 1 cup tomato sauce

- 3/4 head iceberg lettuce - rinsed, dried, and shredded
- 2 tomatoes, chopped
- 1 (16 ounce) package corn chips

Directions

Place beef, onion, bell pepper, garlic, and cumin in a large, deep skillet. Cook over medium-high heat until the hamburger is evenly brown. Drain any excess fat.

Stir cheese, green chilies, and tomato sauce into the beef mixture. Cook for 5 minutes, or until cheese is melted.

Equally, divide lettuce among salad plates. Pour meat and cheese mixture over lettuce and garnish with chopped tomato and corn chips.

Mexican Style Cornbread

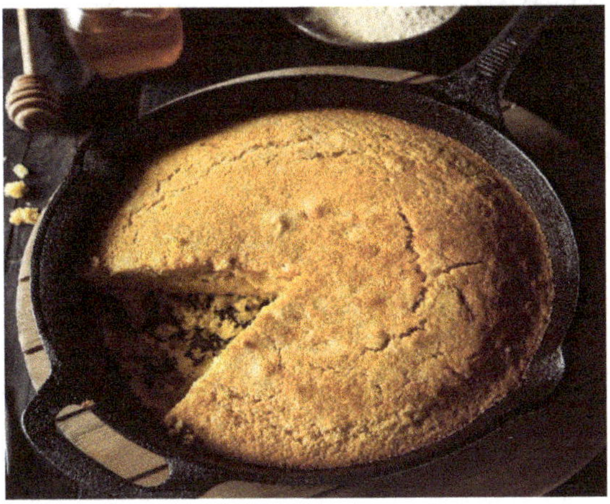

Ingredients

- 2 eggs
- 1/4 cup corn oil 1 cup buttermilk
- 1 1/2 cups shredded Cheddar cheese
- 1 (8 ounce) can cream-style corn
- 1 large onion, chopped
- 2 fresh jalapeno peppers, seeded and minced
- 1 cup cornmeal
- 1/2 cup all-purpose flour
- 2 teaspoons baking powder
- 1/2 teaspoon baking soda
- 1/2 teaspoon salt

Directions

Preheat oven to 350 degrees F (175 degrees C). Grease an 8-inch square baking dish or a cast-iron skillet.

In a small bowl, beat eggs. Mix in corn oil and buttermilk. Stir in 1 cup shredded cheese, creamed corn, onion, and jalapenos.

In a large bowl, whisk together cornmeal, flour, baking powder, soda, and salt. Stir the egg mixture into the dry ingredients. Mix well. Pour batter into prepared pan. Sprinkle remaining 1/2 cup cheese on top.

Bake for 30 to 35 minutes until the center is set and the top is golden brown.

Mexican Cornbread II

Ingredients

- 1 (8.5 ounce) package self-rising cornmeal
- 1 egg
- 1/2 cup milk
- 1 (8 ounce) can cream-style corn
- 1 cup shredded Monterey Jack cheese
- 1 (4 ounce) can diced green chile peppers, drained

Directions

Preheat oven to 400 degrees F (200 degrees C). Lightly grease a 9x9 inch baking pan.

Place cornmeal mix in a large bowl. Stir in egg, milk, creamed corn, cheese, and diced green chile peppers. Spread batter into prepared pan.

Bake in preheated oven for 25 minutes, or until golden brown and cornbread pulls away from sides of the pan.

Mexican Turkey

Ingredients

- 1 teaspoon vegetable oil
- 1 onion, chopped
- 1-pound shredded cooked turkey
- 1 teaspoon garlic powder
- 1 large fresh tomato, chopped
- 1/2 cup water
- 1 tablespoon chopped fresh cilantro
- salt and pepper to taste

Directions

Heat the oil in a skillet over medium heat and cook the onion until tender. Mix in turkey, and season with garlic powder. Stir in the tomato. Pour in water, sprinkle with cilantro, and season with salt and pepper. Cover skillet, and simmer 5 minutes, or until heated through.

Smothered Mexican Lasagna

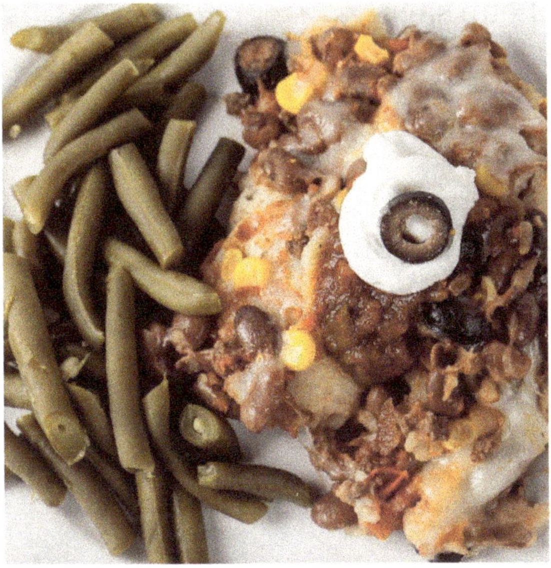

Ingredients

- 1 1/2 pounds ground turkey
- 1 bunch green onions, chopped
- 1 (1.25 ounce) package taco seasoning mix
- 2 cups water
- 1 (14.5 ounce) can diced tomatoes, undrained
- 1 (4 ounce) can diced green chile peppers, undrained
- 1 (15 ounce) container ricotta cheese
- 2 eggs

- 8 (10 inch) flour tortillas
- 1 (8 ounce) container sour cream
- 1/4 cup salsa

Directions

Preheat oven to 400 degrees F (200 degrees C). Place ground turkey in a large, deep skillet. Cook over medium-high heat until evenly brown. Stir in green onions, taco seasoning mix, water, diced tomatoes with juice, and green chiles with juice. Reduce heat to medium.

In a medium bowl, mix together ricotta and eggs. Place 2 tortillas in the bottom of a 9x13 inch pan. Spread 1/4 of the ricotta mixture on tortillas. Spoon 1/4 of the meat mixture over the cheese. Repeat layers until all is used up.

Bake in preheated oven for 20 minutes, or until sauce is bubbly. In a small bowl, mix together sour cream and salsa. Serve in a bowl on the side.

Mexican Casserole

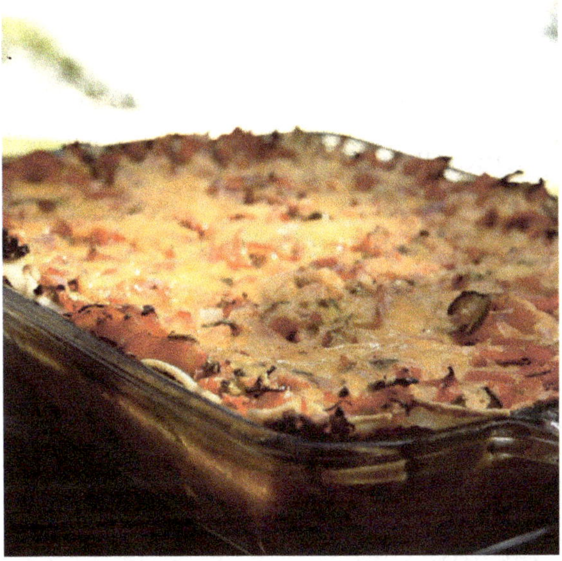

Ingredients

- 1 (16 ounce) can refried beans
- 3/4 onion, diced
- 5 (10 inch) flour tortillas
- 1 cup salsa
- 2 cups shredded Cheddar or Colby Jack cheese

Directions

Preheat oven to 375 degrees F (190 degrees C). Spray a 9-inch pie pan with non-stick cooking spray.

In a saucepan, cook refried beans and onions (to soften them) on medium-high heat for about 5 minutes.

Place one tortilla in the bottom of the greased pan. Spread about 1/3 cup of the bean mixture over it. Layer a few tablespoons of salsa over this. Then, place another tortilla over the salsa, and add more of the bean mixture. Follow the beans with a big handful of cheese, spreading evenly. Repeat layers, spreading the ingredients evenly over the tortillas. On the top layer, make sure to use lots of salsa and cheese!

Bake until the cheese is melted, approximately 15 to 20 minutes.

Austin Margarita (aka Mexican Martini)

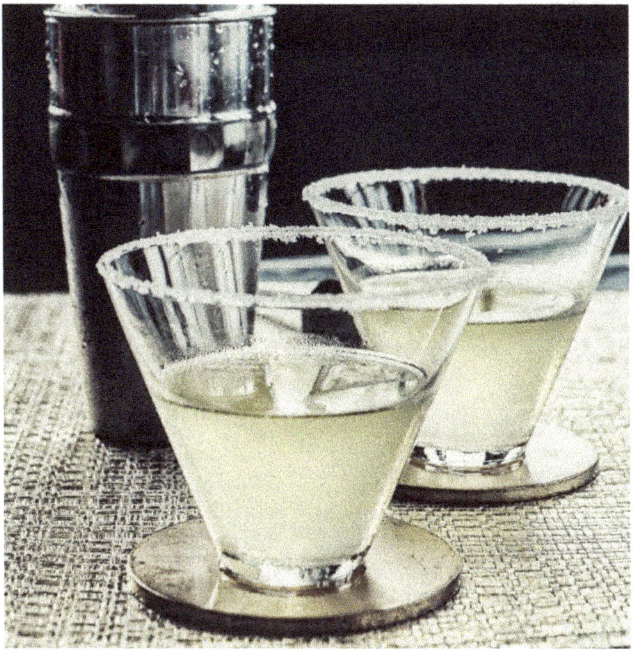

Ingredients

- 1/2 cup ice cubes
- 1 (1.5 fluid ounce) jigger silver tequila
- 1 (1.5 fluid ounce) jigger Cointreau
- 2 teaspoons Grand Marnier liqueur (optional)
- 2 (1.5 fluid ounce) jiggers freshly squeezed lime juice

- 1 (1.5 fluid ounce) jigger freshly squeezed orange juice
- 1 (1.5 fluid ounce) jigger freshly squeezed lemon juice
- 3 pimento-stuffed green olives (optional)

Directions

Place the ice cubes into a margarita glass. Pour in the tequila, Cointreau, and Grand Marnier. Pour in the lime juice, orange juice, and lemon juice to taste. Garnish with a pimento-stuffed olive if desired.

Mexican White Rice

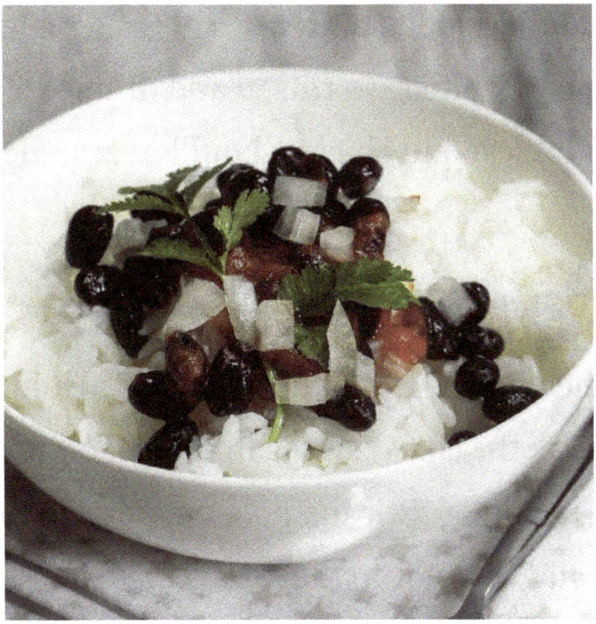

Ingredients

- 1 tablespoon vegetable oil
- 1/2 cup fresh corn kernels
- 1 fresh poblano chile pepper - seeded, deveined, and chopped
- 1/2 onion, chopped
- 1/4 cup drained canned peas
- 1 clove garlic, minced
- 1/4 cup minced carrot

- 1 cup water
- 1 cup milk
- 2 tablespoons butter
- 1 cup white rice, rinsed and drained
- 1 tablespoon chicken bouillon granules

Directions

Heat the oil in a large saucepan over medium-high heat; cook the corn kernels in the hot oil until tender, about 5 minutes. Stir the poblano pepper, onion, peas, garlic, and carrot into the corn; cook and stir for another 5 minutes.

Pour the water and milk into the mixture; bring to a boil. Allow the butter to melt into the boiling mixture. Add the rice and stir. Season with chicken bouillon; cover the saucepan, reduce heat to medium-low, and simmer the mixture until all the liquid is absorbed and the rice is tender for about 20 minutes.

Scrumptious 5-Layer Mexican Dip

Ingredients

- 1 (15.5 ounce) can refried black beans
- 1 tablespoon chili powder
- 1/2 teaspoon ground cumin
- 1 cup KNUDSEN Sour Cream
- 1 cup shredded Cheddar cheese
- 3 green onions, sliced
- 1/3 cup sliced black olives
- 1 tomato, chopped

Directions

Mix beans, chili powder, and cumin; spread onto bottom of 9-inch pie plate.

Top with layers of remaining ingredients.

Refrigerate for several hours or until chilled. Serve with tortilla chips.

Mexican Lasagna Chip Dip

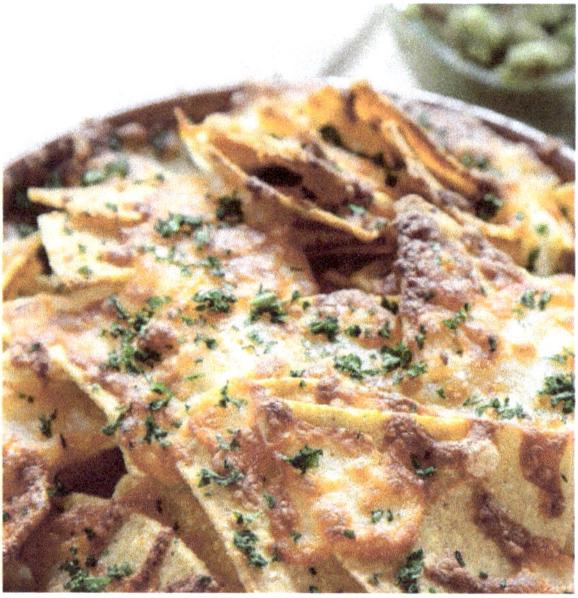

Ingredients

- 1 pound ground beef
- 1 cup diced onion
- 1 (16 ounce) jar salsa
- 2 (16 ounce) cans refried beans
- 2 (4 ounce) cans chopped green chile peppers
- 1 (2 ounce) can sliced black olives, drained
- 2 (8 ounce) packages cream cheese, sliced
- 2 cups shredded Cheddar cheese

Directions

Preheat oven to 400 degrees F (200 degrees C).

Place ground beef and onions in a large, deep skillet. Cook over medium-high heat until onions are soft and ground beef is evenly brown. Remove from heat.

Drain beef and mix in salsa, refried beans, green chile peppers, and black olives. Transfer mixture to a 9x13 inch baking dish. Layer with cream cheese slices. Top with Cheddar cheese.

Bake in the preheated oven for 10 to 15 minutes or until cheese is melted.

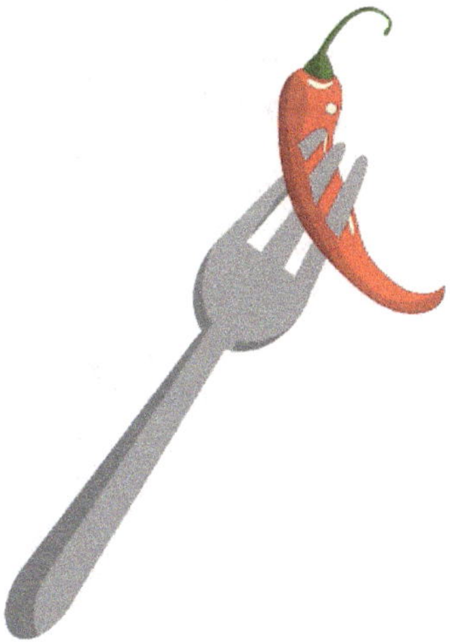

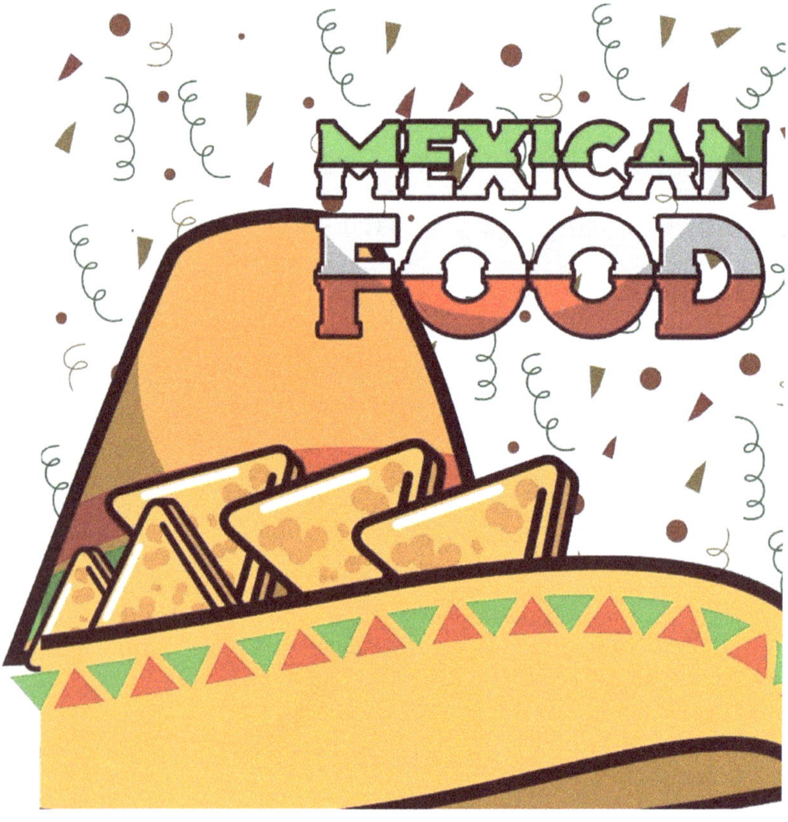
MEXICAN
FOOD

Mexican Lasagna

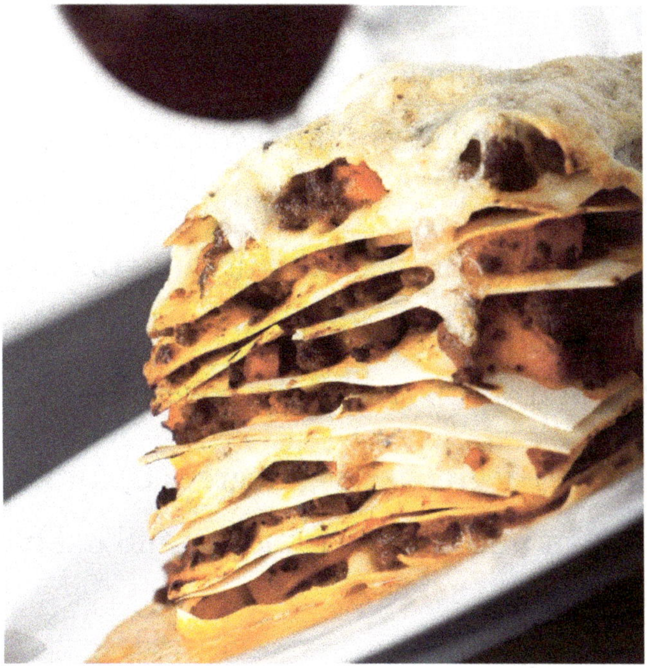

Ingredients

- 1-pound lean ground beef
- 1 (1 ounce) package taco seasoning mix
- 1 (14 ounce) can of peeled and diced tomatoes with juice
- 10 (6 inch) corn tortillas
- 1 cup prepared salsa
- 1/2 cup shredded Colby cheese

Directions

Preheat oven to 350 degrees F (175 degrees C).

In a large skillet over medium-high heat, brown the ground beef, and stir in the taco seasoning and tomatoes. Line a 9x13-inch baking dish with half the tortillas. Spoon the beef mixture into the dish, then top with the remaining tortillas. Spread salsa over the tortillas and sprinkle with the cheese.

Bake at 350 degrees F (175 degrees C) for 20 to 30 minutes, or until cheese is melted and bubbly

Mexican Lasagna (1)

Ingredients

- 1-pound extra-lean ground beef
- 1 (16 ounce) can refried beans
- 2 teaspoons dried oregano
- 1 teaspoon ground cumin
- 3/4 teaspoon garlic powder
- 12 dry lasagna noodles
- 1/2 cups water
- 2 1/2 cups salsa
- 2 cups sour cream
- 3/4 cup chopped green onions
- 1 (2 ounce) can sliced black olives
- 1 cup shredded Pepper Jack cheese

Directions

In a large skillet, cook the ground beef over medium-high heat until evenly brown. Drain off excess fat. In a large bowl, combine the cooked beef, refried beans, oregano, cumin, and garlic powder.

Place four of the uncooked lasagna noodles in the bottom of a 9x13 inch baking dish. Spread half of the beef mixture over the noodles. Top with 4 more uncooked noodles and the remaining half of the beef mixture. Cover with remaining noodles. Combine the water and the salsa in a medium bowl and pour it overall.

Cover tightly with foil. Bake at 350 degrees F (175 degrees C) for 1 1/2 hours, or until noodles are tender.

In a medium bowl, combine the sour cream, green onions, and olives. Spoon over casserole and top with shredded cheese. Return to the oven, and bake for an additional 5 to 10 minutes, or until cheese is melted.

Mexican Lasagna (2)

Ingredients

- 1-pound lean ground beef
- 1 (1.25 ounce) package taco seasoning mix
- 2 (16 ounce) cans refried beans
- 4 (10 inch) flour tortillas
- 3 cups shredded Cheddar cheese
- 2 green onions, chopped
- 2 roma (plum) tomatoes, chopped

Directions

Preheat oven to 375 degrees F (190 degrees C).

In a large skillet over medium heat, cook beef until browned. Drain. Combine with taco seasoning and refried beans. Spread half of the mixture in a 9x13 inch baking dish. Top with two tortillas, trimming if necessary, and half of the cheese. Repeat layers.

Bake 35 to 45 minutes until heated through and cheese is bubbly. Top with green onions and tomatoes. Let cool 5 minutes before serving.

Mexican Lasagna Rollups

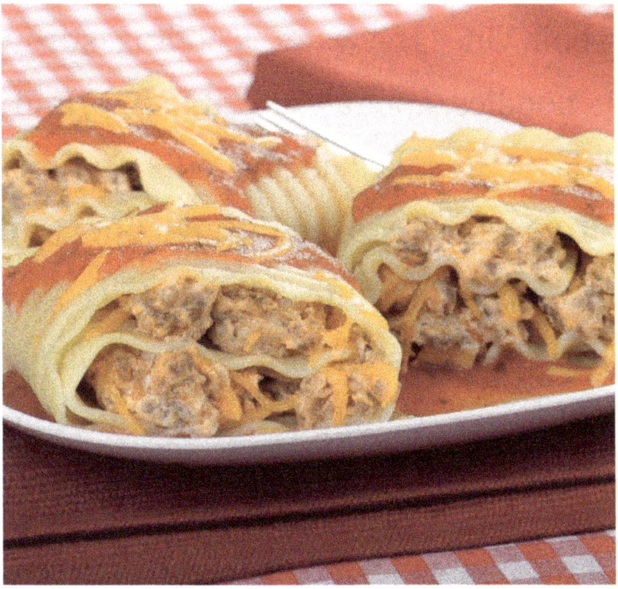

Ingredients

- 10 uncooked lasagna noodles
- 1 (16 ounce) jar salsa
- 1 pound ground beef
- 1 (1 ounce) packet taco seasoning mix
- 1 (16 ounce) package cottage cheese
- 1/2 cup grated Parmesan cheese
- 1 (15.5 ounce) jar prepared salsa con queso sauce
- 1 1/2 cups shredded Mexican cheese blend

Directions

Fill a large pot with lightly salted water and bring to a rolling boil. Once the water is boiling, stir in the lasagna noodles, about 3 or 4 at a time, and return to a boil. Cook the noodles uncovered, occasionally stirring, until the pasta has cooked through but is still firm to the bite, about 10 minutes per batch. Drain well in a colander set in the sink, and lay the cooked noodles flat on waxed paper or aluminum foil while you finish cooking the rest of the noodles.

Preheat oven to 375 degrees F (190 degrees C). Grease a 9x13-inch baking dish and spread the salsa evenly over the bottom of the dish.

Place the ground beef in a skillet over medium heat, sprinkle with taco seasoning, and cook and stir the meat, breaking it up as it cooks, until the meat is browned and crumbly, about 10 minutes. Drain the fat and place the meat in a large bowl.

Mix cottage cheese and Parmesan cheese into the meat. Place a cooked lasagna noodle out flat and spread about 1/3 cup of the cheese and meat mixture along the length of the noodle. Roll up the noodle, and place the filled rolls, seam sides down, into the prepared baking dish. Spoon about 1 1/2 tablespoons of the queso sauce over each roll. Cover the dish with aluminum foil.

Bake in the preheated oven until the sauce is hot and bubbling for about 40 minutes. Uncover the dish and spread the Mexican cheese blend over the rolls. Return to the oven, and bake until the cheese is melted 8 to 10 more minutes.

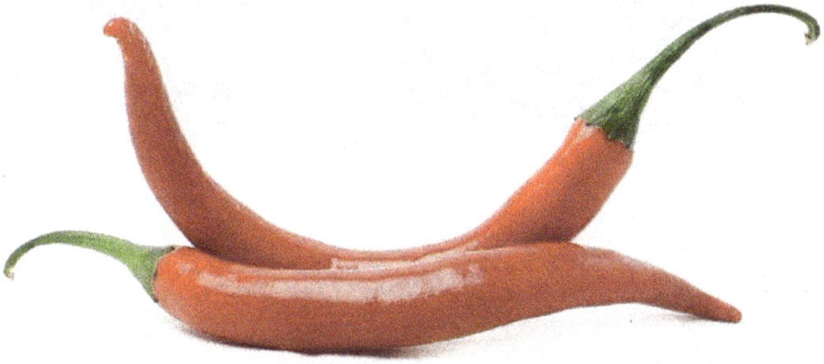

Mexican Egg Rolls

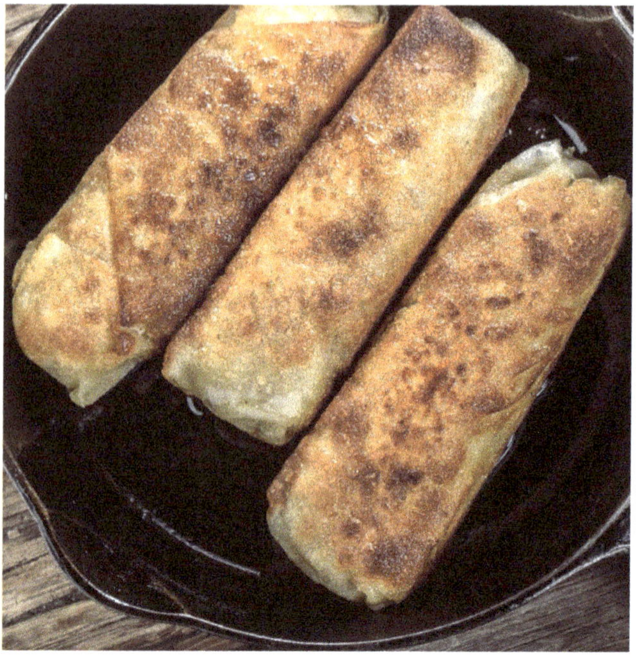

Ingredients

- 1 (14 ounce) package egg roll wrappers
- 1-pound lean ground beef
- 1 (1.25 ounce) package taco seasoning mix
- 1 (4 ounce) can diced green chilies, drained
- 2 cups shredded pepper jack cheese
- 4 cups oil for frying, or as needed

Directions

Crumble ground beef into a large skillet over medium-high heat. Cook until evenly browned and drain off grease. Add taco seasoning and cook according to package directions. Set aside.

Heat 1 inch of oil in a large skillet or preheat a deep fryer to 375 degrees F (190 degrees C).

Layout one egg roll wrapper at a time and place a little more than a tablespoon of the ground beef in the center. Top with a small spoonful of green chilies and a little bit of shredded cheese. Roll up according to package instructions, and seal edges, wetting with water if necessary. Repeat with remaining wrappers and filling.

Fry the rolls in the hot oil until golden brown on all sides, about 5 minutes. Remove from the oil to drain on paper towels. Serve hot and fresh.

Mexican Orange Chicken

Ingredients

- 8 chicken drumsticks
- 8 chicken thighs
- salt and black pepper to taste
- 1 1/2 cups cubed cooked ham
- 1 1/2 cups canned pineapple chunks
- 1 (12 ounce) package bacon slices, cut into 2-inch pieces 1/2 cup raisins (optional)
- 8 cups freshly squeezed orange juice
- 1/4 cup chicken bouillon granules
- 1/4 cup butter, cut into small chunks

Directions

Preheat an oven to 400 degrees F (200 degrees C). Grease a 9x12- inch baking dish with a cover.

Place the chicken drumsticks and thighs in the prepared baking dish, and sprinkle with salt and pepper. Evenly distribute the ham, pineapple chunks, bacon, and raisins over the chicken.

Stir together the orange juice and chicken bouillon granules in a bowl and pour the mixture over the top of the dish. Dot the top evenly with chunks of butter.

Cover, and bake in the preheated oven until the chicken is very tender and the sauce has started to reduce about 1 1/2 hours. Uncover, baste the chicken pieces with the juices in the bottom of the pan, and return to the oven until the chicken is golden for about 30 more minutes.

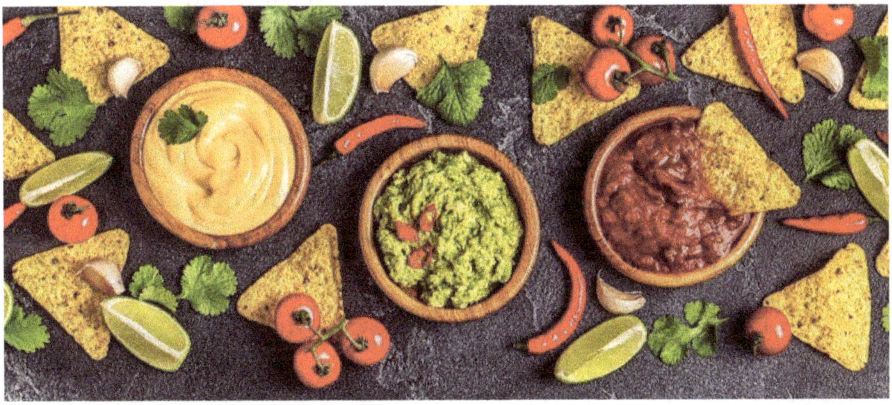

Absolute Mexican Cornbread

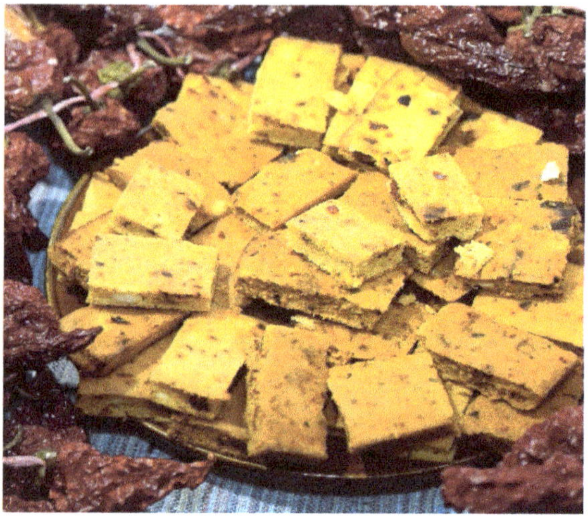

Ingredients

- 1 cup butter, melted 1 cup white sugar
- 4 eggs
- 1 (15 ounce) can cream-style corn
- 1/2 (4 ounce) can chopped green chile peppers, drained
- 1/2 cup shredded Monterey Jack cheese
- 1/2 cup shredded Cheddar cheese
- 1 cup all-purpose flour 1 cup yellow cornmeal
- 4 teaspoons baking powder
- 1/4 teaspoon salt

Directions

Preheat oven to 300 degrees F (150 degrees C). Lightly grease a 9x13 inch baking dish.

In a large bowl, beat together butter and sugar. Beat in eggs one at a time. Blend in cream corn, chiles, Monterey Jack, and Cheddar cheese.

In a separate bowl, stir together flour, cornmeal, baking powder, and salt. Add flour mixture to corn mixture; stir until smooth. Pour batter into prepared pan.

Bake in preheated oven for 1 hour, until a toothpick inserted into the center of the pan, comes out clean.

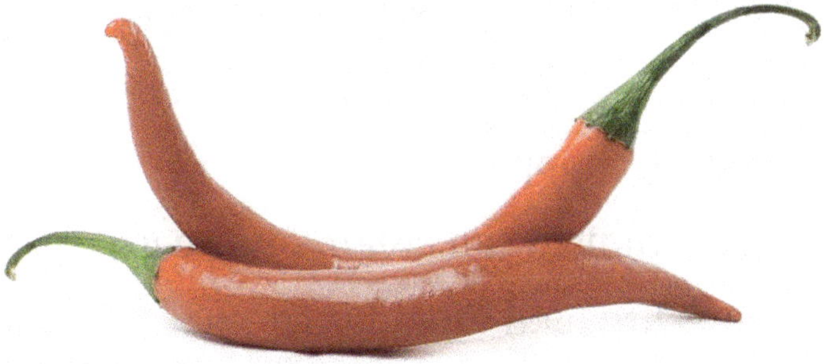

Mom's Mexican Cornbread

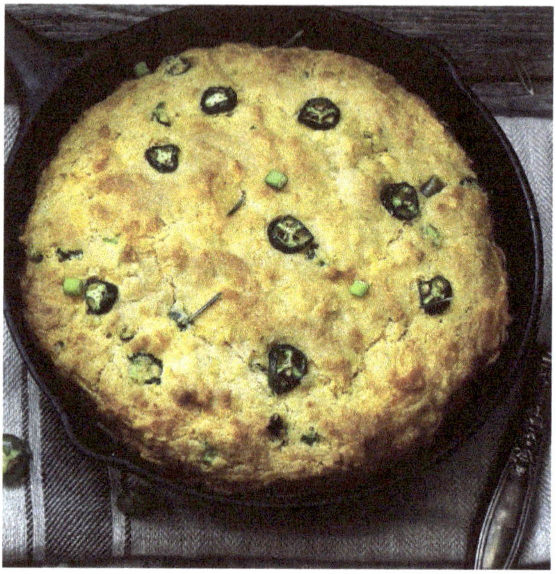

Ingredients

- 1 pound ground beef 1 cup cornmeal
- 1 teaspoon salt
- 1 teaspoon baking soda 1 cup milk
- 1 egg
- 1 onion, chopped
- 1 (14.5 ounce) can cream-style corn
- 1 cup shredded Cheddar cheese
- 2 jalapeno peppers, chopped

Directions

Preheat an oven to 350 degrees F (175 degrees C). Coat a 9x12 inch baking dish with cooking spray.

Heat a large skillet over medium heat; cook the ground beef in the skillet until no longer pink. Set aside.

In a large bowl, stir together the cornmeal, salt, and baking soda. Mix in milk, egg, onion, corn, Cheddar cheese, and jalapeno pepper. Stir in browned beef. Pour into the prepared baking dish.

Bake in the preheated oven until golden brown, about 1 hour.

Mexican Style Meatballs

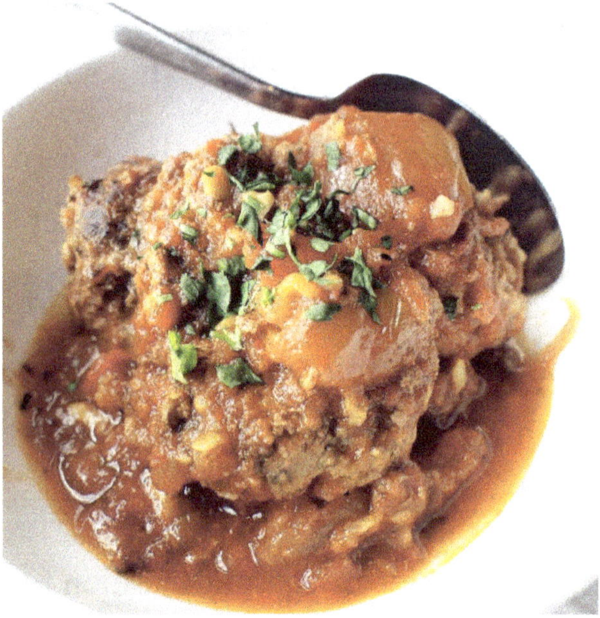

Ingredients

- 1 1/2 pounds ground beef
- 1 1/2 pounds ground pork
- 2 eggs
- 1 1/2 cups plain dried breadcrumbs
- 1 teaspoon salt
- 1 teaspoon ground black pepper
- 2 cloves garlic, minced
- 1/2 cup water

- 2 (28 ounce) cans diced tomatoes with juice
- 3 chipotle peppers in adobo sauce
- 4 teaspoons vegetable oil
- 2 small onions, minced
- 4 cloves garlic, minced
- 2 teaspoons ground cumin
- 2 cups chicken broth
- 1 teaspoon salt
- 1/2 cup chopped fresh cilantro for garnish (optional)

Directions

In a large bowl, mix together the ground beef and pork, eggs, breadcrumbs, 1 teaspoon of salt, pepper, 2 cloves of minced garlic, and water using your hands. Form into 1-inch meatballs and set aside on a piece of waxed paper.

Pour the diced tomatoes into the container of a blender along with the chipotle peppers. Blend until smooth and set aside.

Heat the oil in a large Dutch oven over medium heat. Add the onion; cook, and stir until tender. Stir in the remaining garlic and cumin and cook for a few minutes to release the aromas. Pour in the tomato mixture and chicken broth. Season with the remaining teaspoon of salt and mix well. Bring to a boil, then simmer over low heat while you brown the meatballs.

Heat a large skillet over medium-high heat. Spray with cooking spray. Add meatballs, but do not crowd them. Fry them in two batches if necessary. Cook, occasionally stirring until browned on the outside. Remove from the skillet, and place into the pot of simmering sauce. Let the meatballs simmer in the sauce for about 30 minutes. Longer will not hurt them.

For special occasions, serve the meatballs in a chafing dish with the sauce, and garnish with cilantro.

Basic Mexican Guacamole

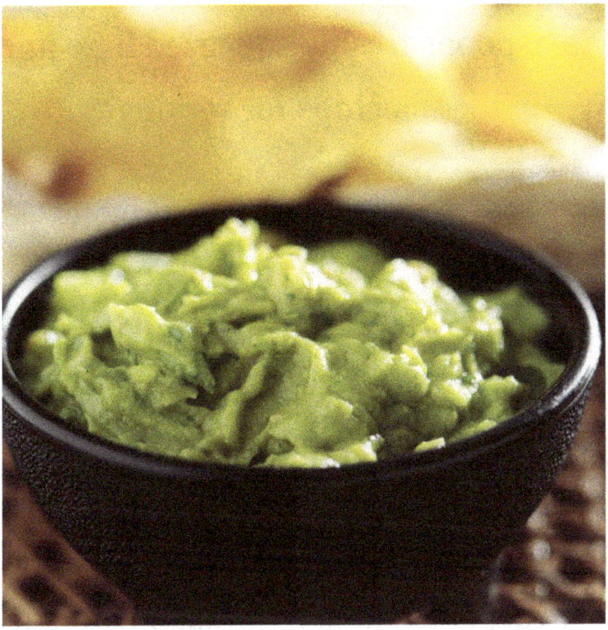

Ingredients

- 2 tablespoons finely chopped fresh cilantro leaves
- 2 teaspoons finely chopped yellow onions
- 2 teaspoons minced jalapeno or Serrano chilies, seeds and membranes removed, if desired Kosher or coarse salt
- 2 large ripe Avocados, peeled and seeded

- 2 tablespoons cored, seeded, and finely chopped plum tomato
- 2 teaspoons freshly squeezed lime juice
- Warm tortilla chips for serving

Directions

Mash together 1 tablespoon of the cilantro, 1 teaspoon of the onion, 1 teaspoon of the chile, and 1/2 teaspoon of salt in the bottom of a molcajete or medium-sized bowl.

Add the avocados and gently mash with a fork until chunky- smooth. Fold the remaining cilantro, onion, and chile into the mixture.

Stir in the tomato and lime juice, adjust the seasonings to taste, and serve with a basket of warm corn tortilla chips.

Campbell's Kitchen Mexican Stroganoff

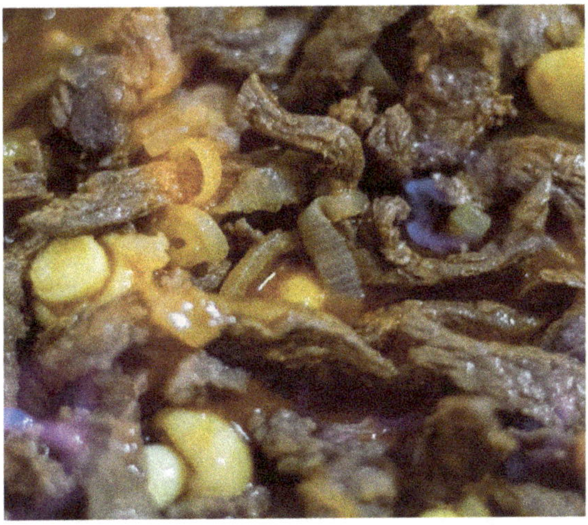

Ingredients

- 2 teaspoons butter
- 1 medium onion, chopped 1 clove garlic, minced
- 1 pound ground beef
- 1 (1 ounce) package taco seasoning mix
- 1 (10.75 ounce) can Campbell'sB® Condensed Cream of Mushroom with Roasted Garlic Soup
- 3/4 cup sour cream
- 1/4 cup PaceB® Picante Sauce Hot cooked egg noodles

Directions

Heat the butter in a 10-inch skillet over medium heat. Add the onion and garlic and cook until tender. Remove the onion mixture from the skillet.

Cook the beef in the skillet over medium-high heat until well browned, often stirring to separate meat. Pour off any fat.

Stir the onion mixture, taco seasoning, soup, sour cream, and Picante sauce in the skillet and cook until the mixture is hot and bubbling, stirring often. Serve the beef mixture over the noodles.

Creamy Mexican Dip

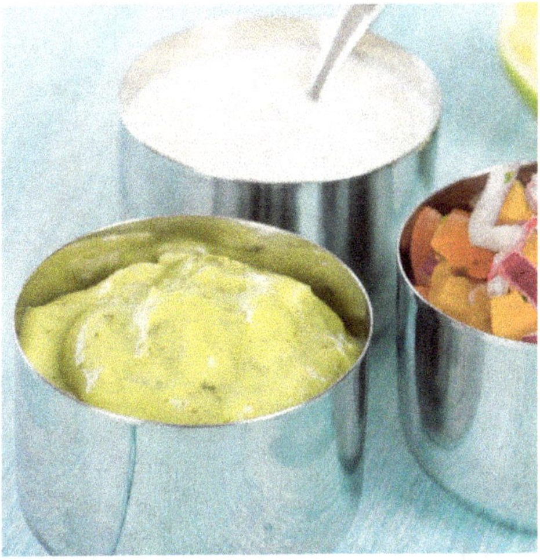

Ingredients

- 1 (16 ounce) container sour cream
- 1 1/2 cups shredded sharp Cheddar cheese
- 1/2 cup salsa
- 1 avocado - peeled, pitted, and diced

Directions

In a medium-size bowl, combine sour cream, Cheddar cheese, salsa, and avocado. Combine ingredients until they are just mixed. Cover and chill until you are ready to serve.

Easy Mexican Casserole

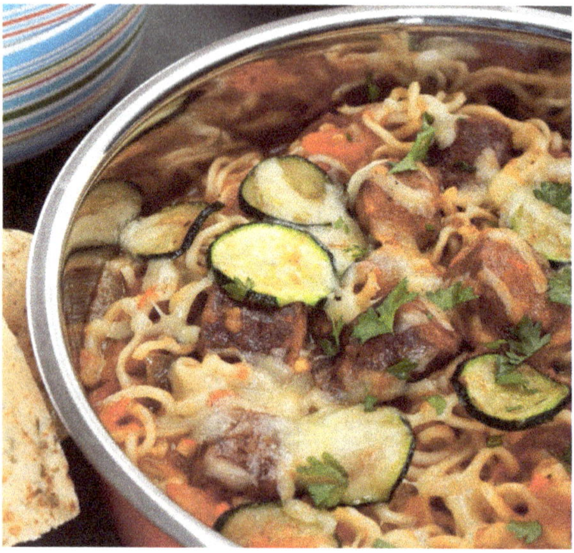

Ingredients

- 1-pound lean ground beef
- 2 cups salsa
- 1 (16 ounce) can chili beans, drained
- 3 cups tortilla chips, crushed
- 2 cups sour cream
- 1 (2 ounce) can sliced black olives, drained
- 1/2 cup chopped green onion
- 1/2 cup chopped fresh tomato
- 2 cups shredded Cheddar cheese

Directions

Preheat oven to 350 degrees F (175 degrees C).

In a large skillet over medium-high heat, cook ground beef until no longer pink. Stir in salsa, reduce heat, and simmer 20 minutes, or until liquid is absorbed. Stir in beans, and heat through.

Spray a 9x13 baking dish with cooking spray. Spread crushed tortilla chips in the dish, and then spoon beef mixture over chips. Spread sour cream over beef, and sprinkle olives, green onion, and tomato over the sour cream. Top with Cheddar cheese.

Bake in preheated oven for 30 minutes, or until hot and bubbly.

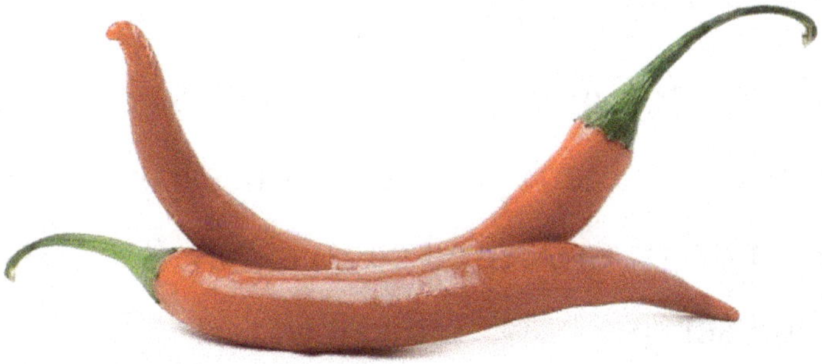

Mexican Salsa II

Ingredients

- 5 roma (plum) tomatoes
- 3 serrano peppers
- 1/2 cup chopped onion
- 2/3 cup chopped fresh cilantro
- 1 clove garlic, peeled and crushed salt to taste

Directions

Place roma (plum) tomatoes and serrano peppers in a medium saucepan over medium-high heat with enough water to cover. Bring to a boil. Boil 15 minutes. Remove from heat and drain.

Place roma tomatoes, serrano peppers, onion, cilantro, and garlic in a blender or food processor. Puree about 30 seconds, or to desired consistency. Transfer to a medium serving bowl and salt to taste.

Mexican Posole Stew

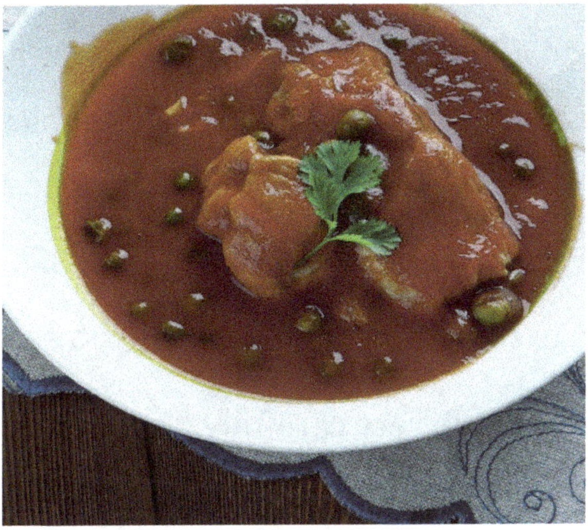

Ingredients

- 2 pounds boneless pork loin, cubed
- 8 ounces fried pork skins
- 2 pig's feet
- 1 tablespoon salt
- 2 (15 ounce) cans white hominy, drained
- 1 tcaspoon dried oregano
- 2 cloves garlic, crushed
- 2 tablespoons chopped onion
- 4 dried hot red chile pepper pods, seeded and diced

Directions

Place meat, pork rinds, and pork shanks in a large kettle and add about 5 quarts of water or enough to cover the meat. Add approximately 1 tablespoon salt and bring to a boil. Cook over medium heat for about 1 1/2 hours.

Remove excess grease and set aside. Reserve liquid.

Wash the posole very carefully until the water is clear so as to remove lime from kernels. Put in a large kettle and cover with water. Boil until posole has popped.

Mix meat, posole, rind, and shanks or pigs' feet. Add oregano, garlic, onion, and chile pods. Let simmer for about 1/2 hour.

Caldo de Res (Mexican Beef Soup)

Ingredients

- 1/4 cup sliced pickled jalapenos
- 1/4 cup finely chopped onion
- 1 cup chopped fresh cilantro
- 2 limes, cut into wedges
- 4 radishes, quartered

Directions

Cut the meat from the beef bones into about 1/2-inch pieces, leaving some on the bones.

Heat a heavy soup pot over medium-high heat until very hot. Add the oil, tilting the pan to coat the bottom. Add the meat and bones, and season with salt and pepper. Cook and stir until thoroughly browned.

Add 1 onion and cook until onion is also lightly browned. Stir in the tomatoes and broth. The liquid should cover the bones by 1/2 inch. If not, add enough water to compensate. Reduce heat to low, and simmer for 1 hour with the lid on loosely. If meat is not tender, continue cooking for another 10 minutes or so.

Pour in the water and return to a simmer. Add the carrot and 1/4 cup cilantro, and cook for 10 minutes, then stir in the potato, corn, and chayote. Simmer until vegetables are tender. Push the cabbage wedges into the soup and cook for about 10 more minutes.

Ladle soup into large bowls, including meat, vegetables, and bones. Garnish with jalapenos, minced onion, and additional cilantro.

Squeeze lime juice over all and serve with radishes.

Chocolate Mexican Wedding Cookies

Ingredients

- 1 cup butter, softened
- 1/3 cup confectioners' sugar
- 2 teaspoons vanilla extract
- 1 3/4 cups all-purpose flour
- 1 cup ground pecans
- 1/2 cup German sweet chocolate, grated
- 3/4 teaspoon ground cinnamon
- 1 pinch salt
- 1/2 cup confectioners' sugar
- 1/4 cup German sweet chocolate, grated

Directions

In a large bowl, cream the butter and 1/3 cup confectioner's sugar until light and fluffy. Add the vanilla extract.

In a separate bowl, combine the flour, ground pecans, 1/2 cup ground chocolate, cinnamon, and salt; mix well.

Gradually add the dry ingredients to the creamed mixture. Wrap dough in plastic wrap and chill 1 to 2 hours, or until firm. Preheat oven to 325 degrees F (180 degrees C).

Shape the dough into 1-inch balls. Place balls 1 inch apart on an ungreased baking sheet. Bake 15 to 18 minutes, or until the cookies are firm to the touch. Cool 1 minute on the baking sheet, then transfer to a wire rack.

For the coating, sift 1/2 cup of the confectioner's sugar and 1/4 cup of the ground cocoa into a shallow bowl. While cookies are still warm, roll them in the coating.

Ground Beef Mexican Style

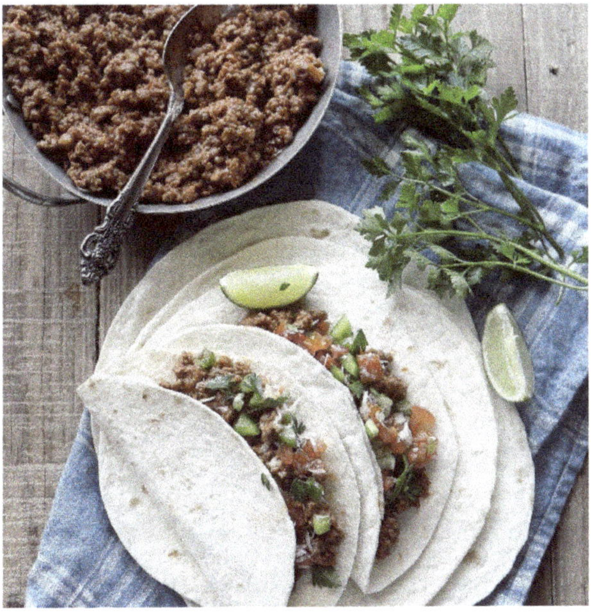

Ingredients

- 1 pound ground beef 1 cup salsa
- 1/2 cup water
- 1 green bell pepper, chopped
- 1 bunch green onions, chopped
- 1 (8 ounce) package wide egg noodles
- 1/2 cup sour cream
- 1/2 cup shredded Cheddar cheese
- 1 tomato, chopped

Directions

In a large nonstick skillet, cook and stir ground beef until browned. Drain off excess fat.

Stir in salsa and water. Simmer for 10 minutes.

Meanwhile, cook pasta in boiling water until al dente. Drain.

Stir in green pepper and onions and continue simmering until veggies are crisp/tender. Stir in noodles and sour cream. Sprinkle grated cheese on top, and cover pan until the cheese melts.

Sprinkle chopped tomatoes on the top and serve.

Hot Mexican Spinach Dip

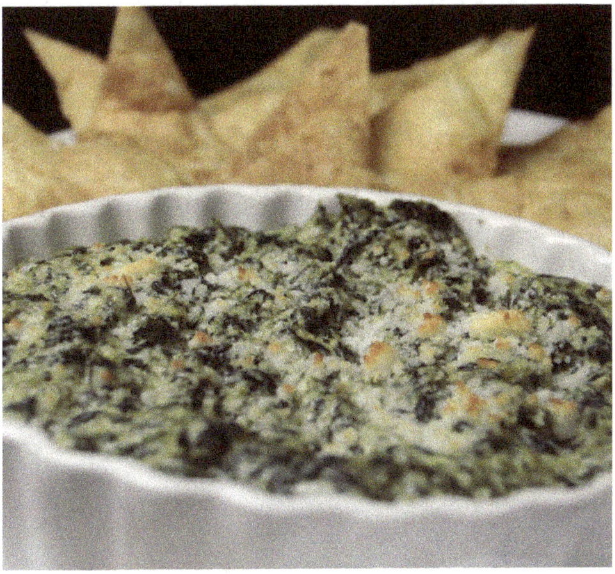

Ingredients

- 1 (16 ounce) jar salsa
- 1 (10 ounce) package frozen chopped spinach, thawed and drained
- 2 cups shredded Monterey Jack cheese
- 1 (8 ounce) package cream cheese, diced and softened 1 cup evaporated milk
- 1 (2.25 ounce) can chopped black olives, drained
- 1 tablespoon red wine vinegar, salt, and pepper to taste

Directions

Preheat oven to 400 degrees F (200 degrees C).

In a medium baking dish, mix together salsa, chopped spinach, Monterey Jack cheese, cream cheese, evaporated milk, black olives, red wine vinegar, salt, and pepper.

Bake mixture in the preheated oven for 12 to 15 minutes, or until bubbly.

Mexican-Style Goulash

Ingredients

- 1-pound lean ground beef 1 cup chopped onion
- 1 (14.5 ounce) can diced tomatoes, undrained
- 1 (8 ounce) can tomato sauce 1 cup fresh or frozen corn 1/2 cup water
- 1 1/4 teaspoons chili powder 1 teaspoon dried oregano 1/2 teaspoon salt
- 2/3 cup uncooked elbow macaroni
- 2/3 cup shredded reduced-fat Cheddar cheese

Directions

In a large nonstick skillet, cook beef and onion over medium heat until meat is no longer pink, drain. Stir in the tomatoes, tomato sauce, corn, water, chili powder, oregano, and salt. Bring to a boil. Add macaroni. Reduce heat; cover, and simmer for 20-25 minutes or until macaroni are tender. Sprinkle with cheese; cover and cook 2-3 minutes longer or until cheese is melted.

Mexican Brunch Tortillas

Ingredients

- 3 Breakfast Patties made with Organic Soy
- 6 eggs
- 1/3 cup fat-free milk
- 1/4 teaspoon pepper
- 1/8 teaspoon salt
- 2 teaspoons butter or margarine
- 3 (8 inch) flour tortillas
- 1/4 cup Low-fat Pepper Jack cheese
- 1/2 medium avocado, pitted, peeled, and chopped
- 1 teaspoon lemon juice
- 1/4 cup salsa

Directions

Cook patties according to package directions. Cut in half.

In a medium bowl, beat eggs with a wire whisk until combined. Whisk in milk, pepper, and salt. In a large skillet, heat butter over medium heat until sizzling. Pour in egg mixture. Cook until the mixture begins to set around the edge. Gently scrape spatula across skillet bottom, allowing uncooked portions to flow underneath. Continue until cooked through but still shiny.

Place tortillas on a baking sheet sprayed with nonstick cooking spray. Spoon eggs onto half of each tortilla. Top with patty pieces.

Sprinkle with cheese. Loosely fold tortillas over cheese. Bake at 350 degrees F for 5 to 6 minutes or until cheese melts.

Meanwhile, toss avocado with lemon juice. Cut filled tortillas in half; place on serving plates. Top with avocado and salsa.

Mexican Spinach Dip

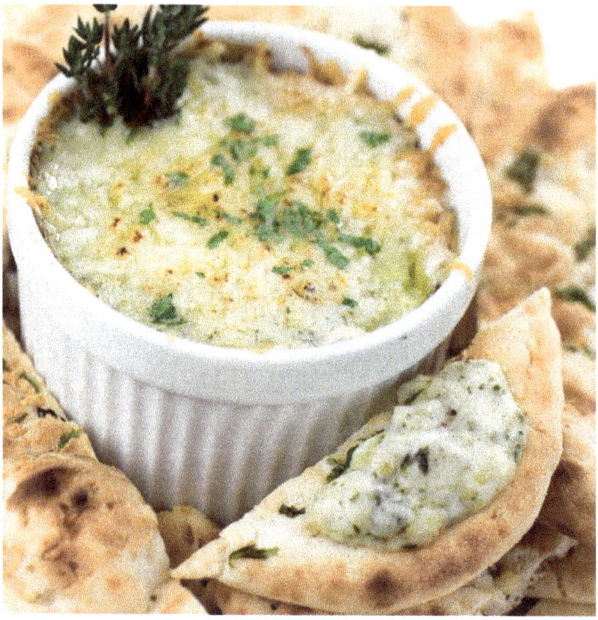

Ingredients

- 8 ounces cream cheese, softened
- 8 ounces sour cream
- 1 (1 pound) loaf processed cheese (i.e., Velveeta®), cubed
- 2 cups shredded Mexican cheese blend
- 2 (10 ounce) cans diced tomatoes with green chile peppers

- 1 (10 ounce) package frozen chopped spinach, thawed and drained
- 1 (1.25 ounce) package taco seasoning mix
- 2 tomatoes, chopped
- 1/2 cup green onions, chopped

Directions

Preheat the oven to 350 degrees F (175 degrees C).

In a 2 quart or 9x13 inch casserole dish, combine the cream cheese, sour cream, and processed cheese. Heat in the microwave until ingredients are soft enough to stir together, about 1 minute.

Stir in the shredded cheese, diced tomatoes with chilies, spinach, and taco seasoning mix. Spread evenly.

Bake uncovered in the preheated oven until hot and bubbly, about 30 minutes. Sprinkle tomatoes and green onions on top before serving. This can also be made ahead of time, refrigerated, and baked just before serving.

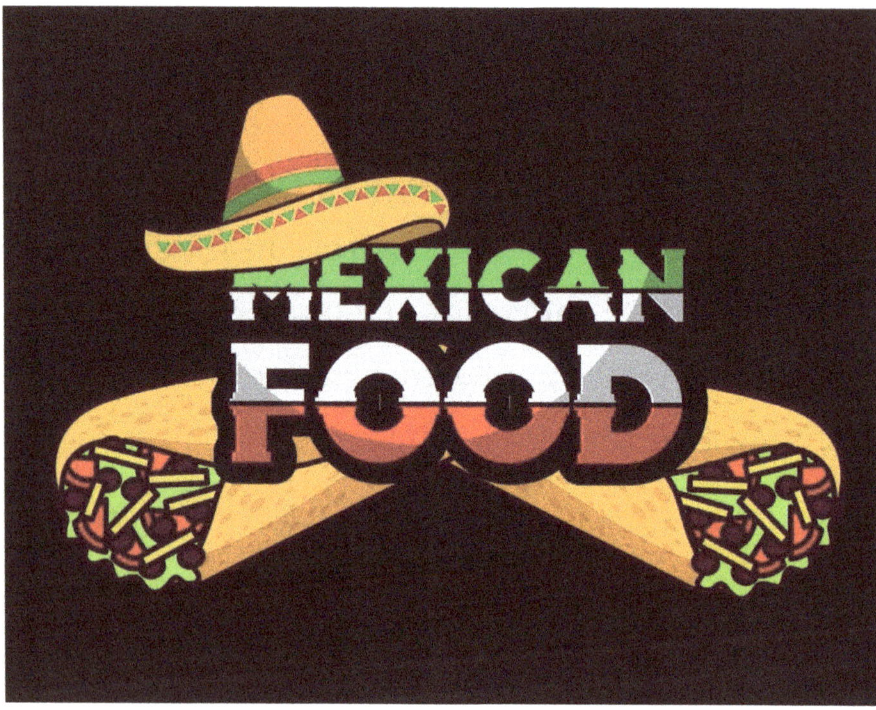
MEXICAN
FOOD

Mexican Grilled Chicken

Ingredients

- 1/2 cup mayonnaise
- 3 tablespoons fresh lime juice
- 1 (1.25 ounce) package taco seasoning mix
- 8 skinless, boneless chicken breast halves

Directions

In a small bowl, mix together mayonnaise, lime juice, and taco seasoning until smooth. Place chicken on grill over medium coals. Sear one side; turn and brush with sauce. Grill, uncovered, for 6 minutes; turn and brush with sauce. Grill another 6 minutes or until chicken juices run clear.

Mexican Chicken and Black Bean Salad

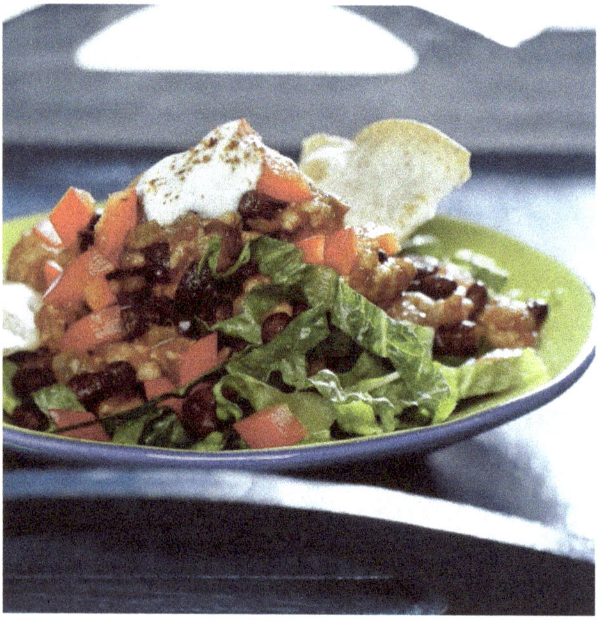

Ingredients

- 2 (4 ounce) frozen skinless, boneless chicken breast halves
- 1 (8 ounce) can low sodium tomato sauce
- 1/4 cup water
- 1 (1 ounce) packet taco seasoning
- 1 (15.5 ounce) can of black beans

- 4 cups baby spinach leaves
- 2 tablespoons fat-free sour cream
- 1/2 cup shredded Mexican cheese blend
- 1/2 cup salsa

Directions

Preheat oven to 375 degrees F (190 degrees C). Lightly grease a baking dish.

Place the chicken breasts in the prepared dish. Mix the tomato sauce, water, and taco seasoning in a small bowl; pour sauce over the chicken.

Bake in preheated oven until chicken is no longer pink in the center, about 30 minutes.

Divide spinach between two plates. Place the chicken breasts on the spinach beds and spoon half the black beans over each piece. Divide sour cream, shredded cheese, and salsa to top each salad.

Mexican Wedding Cakes II

Ingredients

- 1 cup butter, softened
- 8 tablespoons confectioners' sugar
- 2 cups all-purpose flour
- 2 cups chopped walnuts
- 1/2 teaspoon vanilla extract

Directions

Preheat oven to 350 degrees F (180 degrees C).

Mix all the ingredients together with a mixer until well blended. Roll dough into small round balls.

Bake for 10-12 minutes.

Cool completely, then roll in additional confectionary sugar.

Mexican Meat Loaf

Ingredients

- 3/4 cup milk
- 2 eggs, beaten
- 1/2 cup dry breadcrumbs
- 1/4 cup finely chopped onion
- 1/2 teaspoon salt
- 1/2 teaspoon pepper
- 1/2 teaspoon chili powder
- 1 1/2 pounds lean ground beef
- 1 (16 ounce) jar Picante sauce

Directions

In a large bowl, combine the first seven ingredients. Add beef and mix well. Pat into a greased 8-in. x 4-in. x 2-in. loaf pan. Bake, uncovered, at 350 degrees F for 1 hour or until juices run clear; drain. Top with warm Picante sauce.

Mexican Pinto Beans

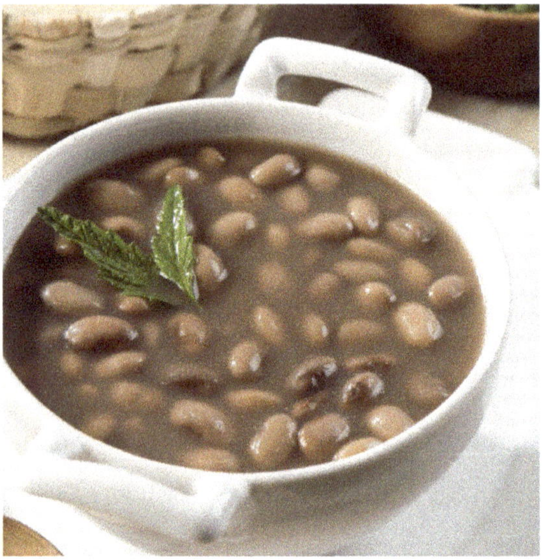

Ingredients

- 1-pound dry pinto beans
- 1/2-pound bacon
- 4 serrano peppers

Directions

Place the beans in a large pot with enough water to cover by 3 to 4 inches and bring to a boil. Remove from heat and let sit 1 hour.

Drain water. Pour in enough fresh water to cover beans by 3 to 4 inches and bring to a boil. Reduce heat, cover, and simmer for 1 hour.

Place bacon in a skillet and cook over medium-high heat until evenly brown. Crumble bacon, and transfer, along with grease, to the pot with the beans. Continue to cook beans on low heat for 30 minutes.

Place the whole chile peppers into the pot, and continue cooking beans for 1 hour, or until tender.

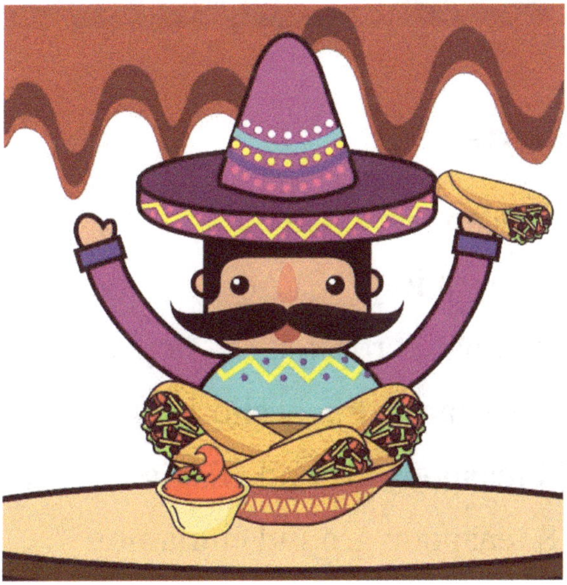

Mexican Salmon

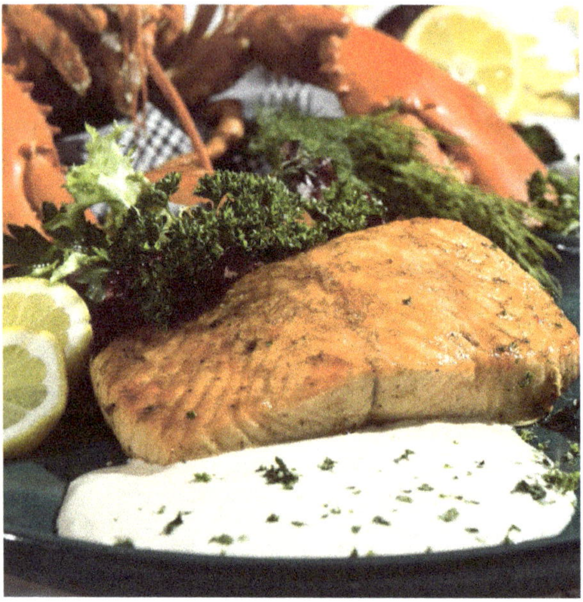

Ingredients

- 2 tablespoons olive oil
- 2 limes, juiced
- 2 marinated roasted red peppers, with liquid
- 1 clove garlic, finely chopped
- 1/8 teaspoon ground allspice
- 1/8 teaspoon ground cinnamon
- 1/4 teaspoon ground cumin
- 1/4 teaspoon white sugar

- salt and pepper to taste
- 1 1/2 pounds salmon steaks
- 1 large tomato, cut into thin wedges
- 3 green onions, chopped
- 1 cup shredded lettuce 1 lime, sliced

Directions

In a medium, nonreactive bowl, mix olive oil, juice of 2 limes, roasted red peppers, garlic, allspice, cinnamon, cumin, sugar, salt, and pepper. Place salmon steaks in a bowl and rub with the mixture. Cover, and marinate in the refrigerator for at least 1 hour.

Preheat the broiler. Arrange salmon steaks on a medium broiler pan, and broil 3 to 5 minutes on each side until the flesh is easily flaked with a fork.

Mix tomato wedges and green onions in a small bowl. Serve salmon with the tomato mixture and lettuce. Garnish with lime wedges.

Mexican Corn Salad

Ingredients

- 3 tablespoons butter
- 2 cups whole corn kernels, cooked
- 1 red bell pepper, diced 1 cup chopped zucchini
- 2 green onions, chopped
- 1 jalapeno pepper, seeded and minced
- 1/2 cup salsa
- 2 tablespoons chopped fresh cilantro

Directions

In a heavy large skillet, melt the butter over medium-high heat. Add the corn, bell pepper, zucchini, green onions, and jalapeno pepper. Saute until vegetables are tender, about 6 minutes. Remove from heat and refrigerate vegetables until chilled.

Add salsa and chopped cilantro to the vegetable mixture. Stir and season with salt and pepper to taste.

Mexican Hot Dip

Ingredients

- 2 (8 ounce) packages cream cheese, softened
- 2 (15 ounce) cans chili
- 1 (6 ounce) can chopped black olives, drained
- 1 (16 ounce) package shredded Cheddar cheese
- 1 green onion, chopped

Directions

Preheat oven to 350 degrees F (175 degrees C).

Spread cream cheese on the bottom of a medium baking dish. Pour in the chili. Spread a layer of olives on the chili, and top with Cheddar cheese and green onion.

Bake uncovered in the preheated oven for 30 minutes or until bubbly and lightly browned.

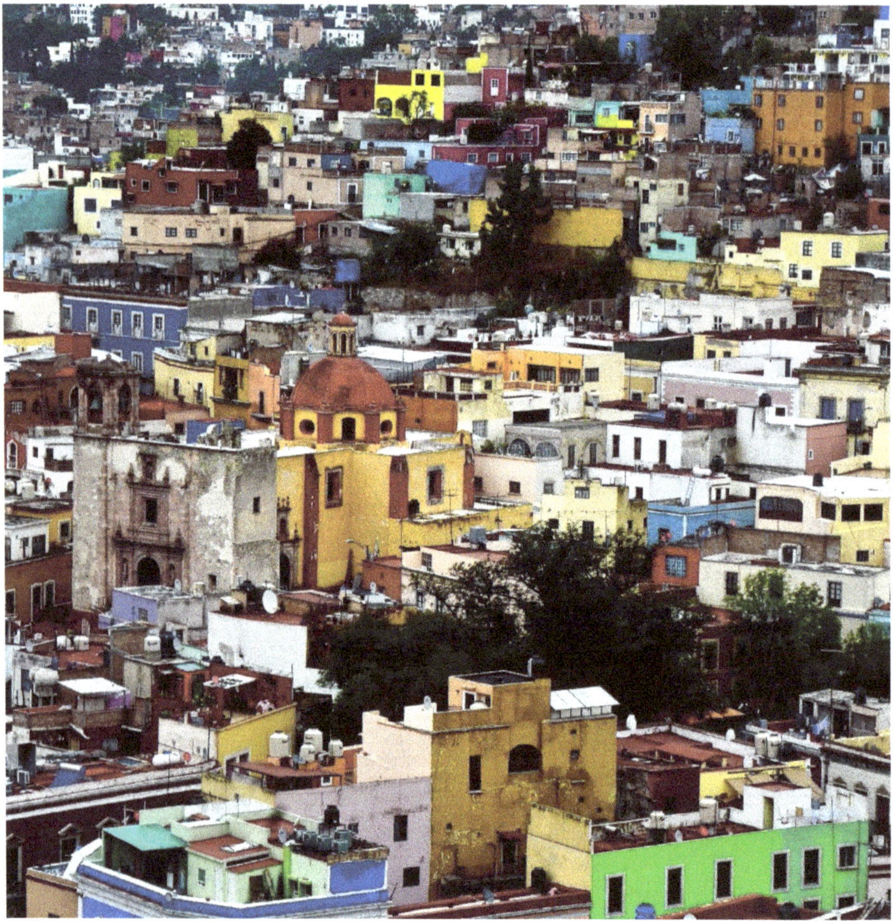